THE *Skinny*
NUTRiBULLET
SUPER GREEN SMOOTHIES
RECIPE BOOK

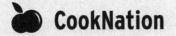 CookNation

THE SKINNY NUTRIBULLET SUPER GREEN SMOOTHIES RECIPE BOOK
DELICIOUS & NUTRITIOUS GREEN SMOOTHIES FOR HEALTHY LIVING & DETOX.

ISBN 978-1-910771-72-3

A CIP catalogue record of this book is available from the British Library

• •

DISCLAIMER

This book is designed to provide information on smoothies and juices that can be made in the NUTRiBULLET appliance only, results may differ if alternative devices are used.

The NutriBullet™ is a registered trademark of Homeland Housewares, LLC. Bell & Mackenzie Publishing is not affiliated with the owner of the trademark and is not an authorized distributor of the trademark owner's products or services.
This publication has not been prepared, approved, or licensed by NutriBullet ™ or Homeland Housewares, LLC.

Some recipes may contain nuts or traces of nuts. Those suffering from any allergies associated with nuts should avoid any recipes containing nuts or nut based oils.
This information is provided and sold with the knowledge that the publisher and author do not offer any legal or other professional advice.
In the case of a need for any such expertise consult with the appropriate professional.
This book does not contain all information available on the subject, and other sources of recipes are available.
This book has not been created to be specific to any individual's or NUTRiBULLET's requirements.
Every effort has been made to make this book as accurate as possible. However, there may be typographical and or content errors. Therefore, this book should serve only as a general guide and not as the ultimate source of subject information.

This book contains information that might be dated and is intended only to educate and entertain.

The author and publisher shall have no liability or responsibility to any person or entity regarding any loss or damage incurred, or alleged to have incurred, directly or indirectly, by the information contained in this book.

CONTENTS

CLEAN & GREEN SMOOTHIES

OTHER COOKNATION TITLES

INTRODUCTION

Just one Nutriblast a day can make a difference to the way you feel and it only takes seconds to make!

WHAT IS A GREEN SMOOTHIE?

Simply speaking a green smoothie is a smoothie which is blended using fresh leafy green vegetables, such as collard greens, kale, chard or spinach. Green herbs such as mint, parsley and coriander are popular too. Most people who advocate the nutritious value of green smoothies believe that its best if the entire smoothie is made from fresh food ingredients. ie: raw fruits rather than frozen or tinned.

WHY ARE GREEN SMOOTHIES SO GOOD FOR YOU?

Leafy green vegetables are some of the most healthy foods on the planet and turning them into smoothies makes them even more digestible and therefore healthier than just eating the greens plain.

GETTING THE BALANCE RIGHT

Green smoothies don't have to be just a blend of 'hardcore' super-greens. In fact with the right mix of ingredients they can be just as tasty as regular smoothies!

If you are experimenting with your own recipes try finding the right balance by starting with less greens, gradually working your way up adding more each time. Alternatively add a little natural sweetener, such as honey or agave nectar: which you can do throughout all the recipes in this book too. You'll also find in general strongly flavored fruits such as mangos & blueberries can sometimes work better than more mild fruits such as bananas and papayas but all have their own plus points so just experiment so suit your own taste.

ABOUT YOUR NUTRIBULLET

If you are reading this you will likely already have purchased a NUTRiBULLET or perhaps are considering buying one. A smart choice! The NUTRiBULLET is unquestionably one of the highest performing smoothie creators on the market. Its clean lines and compact design look great in any kitchen. It's simple to use, easy to clean and the results are amazing.

You may have watched or read some of the NUTRiBULLET marketing videos and literature which make claims of using the power of the NUTRiBULLET to help you lose weight, boost your immune system and fight a number of ailments and diseases. Of course the 'healing' power comes from the foods we use to make our smoothies but the real difference with the NUTRiBULLET is that it EXTRACTS all the goodness of the ingredients. Unlike many juicers and blenders, which leave behind valuable fibre, the NUTRiBULLET pulverizes the food, breaking down their cell walls and unlocking the valuable nutrients so your body can absorb and use them.

You may have made your own smoothies in the past using a blender – you'll know even with a powerful device that there are often indigestible pieces of food left in your glass – not so with the NUTRiBULLET which uses 600 watts to breakdown every part of the food. The manufacturer calls it 'cyclonic action' running at 10,000 revolutions per minute but whatever the marketing jargon, the results speak for themselves.

The NUTRiBULLET is not a blender and not a juicer. It is a nutrient extractor, getting the very best from every ingredient you put in and delivering a nutrient packed Nutriblast. FYI all our recipes make use of the tall cup of the NUTRiBULLET and the extractor blade.

THERE HAS NEVER BEEN A BETTER TIME to introduce health-boosting, weight reducing and well-being green smoothies to your life. With a spiralling obesity epidemic in the western world which in turn is linked to a growing list of debilitating diseases and ailments including diabetes, high blood pressure, heart disease, high cholesterol, infertility, skin conditions and more, the future for many of us can look bleak. Combine this with the super-fast pace of modern life and we can be left feeling fatigued and lethargic, worsened by daily consumption of unhealthy foods.

Using the power from a nutrient packed Nutriblast is an incredibly fast and efficient way of giving our bodies the goodness they need. Making the most of anti-oxidants to protect your cells, omega 3 fatty acids to help your joints, fibre to aid digestion and protein to build and repair muscles.

Just one Nutriblast a day can make a difference to the way you feel and it only takes seconds to make!

The Skinny NUTRiBULLET Green Smoothie Recipe book is packed with delicious and simple recipes. It's so easy to make a green smoothie for a snack or breakfast, and the energy boost and nutrient boost you receive really is palpable.

· ·

Benefits can include:

WEIGHT LOSS · REJUVENATION · GLOWING SKIN · INCREASED ENERGY · LOWER BLOOD PRESSURE · LOWER CHOLESTEROL

and overall enhanced wellbeing.

· ·

TIPS

To help make your Nutriblast fuss-free, follow these quick tips.

· Prepare your shopping list. Take some time to select which Nutriblasts you want to prepare in advance. As
  with all food shopping, make a note of all the ingredients and quantities you need. Depending on the

ingredients it's best not to shop too far in advance to ensure you are getting the freshest produce available. We recommend buying organic produce whenever you can if your budget allows. Organic produce can give a better yield and flavour to your Nutriblast. Remember almost all fruit is fine to freeze too.

- Wash your fruit and veg before juicing. This needn't take up much time but all produce should be washed clean of any traces of bacteria, pesticides and insects.
- To save time prepare produce the night before for early morning Nutriblasts.
- Cut up any produce that may not fit into the tall cup, but only do this just before juicing to keep it as fresh as possible.
- Wash your Nutriblast parts immediately after juicing. As tempting as it may be to leave it till a little later you'll be glad you took the few minutes to rinse and wash before any residue has hardened.
- Substitute where you need to. If you can't source a particular ingredient, try another instead. More often than not you will find the use of a different fruit or veg makes a really interesting and delicious alternative. In our recipes we offer some advice on alternatives but have the confidence to make your own too!
- Some smoothies and juices are sweeter than others. Try drinking these with a straw, you'll find them easier to drink and enjoy.
- Drink lots of water!

IMPORTANT — WHAT NOT TO USE IN YOUR NUTRIBLASTS

The manufacturers of NUTRiBULLET are very clear on the following warning. While the joy of making Nutriblasts is using whole fruit and vegetables there are a few seeds and pits which should be removed. The following contain chemicals which can release cyanide into the body when ingested so do not use any of the following in your Nutriblasts:

- Apple Seeds
- Cherry Pits
- Peach pits
- Apricot Pits
- Plum Pits

CLEANING

Cleaning the NUTRiBULLET is thankfully very easy. The manufacturer gives clear guidelines on how best to do this but here's a recap:

Make sure the NUTRiBULLET is unplugged before disassembling or cleaning.
Set aside the power base and blade holders as these should not be used in a dishwasher.
Use hot soapy water to clean the blades but do not immerse in boiling water as this can warp the plastic.

Use a damp cloth to clean the power base.
All cups and lids can be placed in a dishwasher.
For stubborn marks inside the cup, fill the cup 2/3 full of warm soapy water and screw on the milling blade. Attached to the power base and run for 20-30 seconds.

WARNING:

Do not put your hands or any utensils near the moving blade. Always ensure the NUTRiBULLET is unplugged when assembling/disassembling or cleaning.

ABOUT COOKNATION

CookNation is the leading publisher of innovative and practical recipe books for the modern, health conscious cook.

CookNation titles bring together delicious, easy and practical recipes with their unique approach - easy and delicious, no-nonsense recipes - making cooking for diets and healthy eating fast, simple and fun.

With a range of #1 best-selling titles - from the innovative 'Skinny' calorie-counted series, to the 5:2 Diet Recipes collection - CookNation recipe books prove that 'Diet' can still mean 'Delicious'!

Turn to the end of this book to browse all CookNation's recipe books

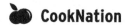 **CookNation**

Skinny

NUTRiBULLET

GREEN BREAKFAST SMOOTHIES

GRAPE, SPINACH & COCONUT SMOOTHIE

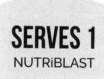

Ingredients

RICH IN FIBRE

- 1 handful seedless green grapes
- 1 handful spinach
- 200ml/7floz light coconut milk
- Handful of ice cubes

Method

1 Rinse the grapes and the spinach well. Remove any thick stalks from the spinach.

2 Add all the ingredients to the NUTRiBULLET tall cup, making sure they do not go past the MAX line on your machine.

3 Just use a few ice cubes to start with until you get the desired consistency.

4 Twist on the NUTRiBULLET blade and blend until smooth.

CHEF'S NOTE

In Sanskrit, the coconut palm is known as kalpa vriksha - 'tree which gives all that is necessary for living.'

12

COCONUT GREEN SMOOTHIE

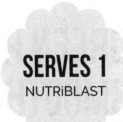
Ingredients

- 175ml/6floz coconut water
- 60ml/2floz coconut milk
- 1 tbsp ground flax seed
- ½ lemon
- ¼ apple

- ¼ orange
- 2 stalks of celery
- Handful of kale
- 3 romaine lettuce leaves

Method

1 Rinse the celery, kale and lettuce. Roughly chop and remove any thick stalks from the kale.

2 Peel and de-seed the lemon and orange. Core the apple.

3 Add all the ingredients to the NUTRiBULLET tall cup, making sure they do not go past the MAX line on your machine.

4 Twist on the NUTRiBULLET blade and blend until smooth.

CHEF'S NOTE

Flax seed are thought to help improve digestion, promote clear skin, lower cholesterol & reduce sugar cravings.

GREEN HONEY MANGO SMOOTHIES

Ingredients

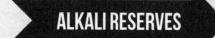

ALKALI RESERVES

- ½ ripe mango
- 1 handful spinach
- 200ml/7 floz light coconut milk
- 2 tbsp plain low-fat yogurt
- 1 tbsp honey

Method

1 Peel and stone the mango.

2 Wash the spinach and remove any thick stalks.

3 Add all the ingredients to the NUTRiBULLET tall cup, making sure they do not go past the MAX line on your machine.

4 Twist on the NUTRiBULLET blade and blend until smooth.

CHEF'S NOTE

Great for breakfast smoothies, low-fat yogurt is not only low in calories, but it also has plenty of beneficial nutrients and probiotics that can boost your overall health.

BLUEBERRY BREAKFAST

Ingredients

BLUEBERRY POWER

- 1 tbsp oats
- 2 handfuls spinach
- 60g/2½oz fresh blueberries
- 200ml/7floz unsweetened almond milk
- 1 tsp agave nectar or honey
- ½-1 tsp grated fresh ginger root
- Water

Method

1 Place the oats in a little water in the NUTRiBULLET tall cup and soak until they have softened (about 15 minutes).

2 Rinse the blueberries and the spinach. Remove any the stalks from the spinach.

3 Add them and the other ingredients to the softened oats, making sure they do not go past the MAX line on your machine (add extra water if you like).

4 Twist on the NUTRiBULLET blade and blend until smooth.

CHEF'S NOTE

Soya milk is also good with this lovely breakfast smoothie. For extra morning energy try adding half a banana.

NUTMEG PUMPKIN SMOOTHIE

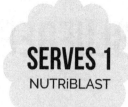

Ingredients

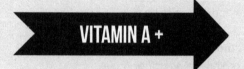

VITAMIN A +

- 200ml/7 floz unsweetened almond milk
- 200g/7oz fresh pumpkin flesh
- 1 handful collared greens
- 1 tbsp honey
- ¼ tsp ground nutmeg
- Water

Method

1 Peel and de-seed the pumpkin.

2 Rinse the collared greens.

3 Add all the ingredients to the NUTRiBULLET tall cup, making sure they do not go past the MAX line on your machine.

4 Only use as much water as you wish to get the consistency right. For a thicker smoothie don't add any at all.

5 Twist on the NUTRiBULLET blade and blend until smooth.

CHEF'S NOTE
Nutmeg contains antioxidants and disease-preventing phytochemicals, some of which are completely unique.

DATE SMOOTHIE

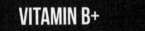

Ingredients

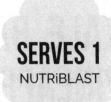

VITAMIN B+

- **175ml/6floz light coconut milk**
- **1 handful pitted dates**
- **1 handful spinach**
- **1 handful kale**
- **Handful of ice cubes**

Method

1 Rinse the spinach & kale and remove any thick stalks.

2 Add all the ingredients to the NUTRiBULLET tall cup. Make sure they do not go past the MAX line on your machine (use as many of the ice cubes as you wish).

3 Twist on the NUTRiBULLET blade and blend until smooth.

CHEF'S NOTE
Fibre rich, dates are easily digested, allowing your body to make full use of their goodness.

KALE, BANANA & PINEAPPLE SMOOTHIE

Ingredients

NUTRIENT DENSE

- 120ml/4 floz light coconut milk
- 1 handful kale
- ¼ pineapple
- 1 banana

Method

1 Rinse the kale and remove any thick stalks.

2 Peel and roughly chop the fresh pineapple.

3 Peel the banana and break into three pieces.

4 Add all the ingredients to the NUTRiBULLET tall cup, making sure they do not go past the MAX line on your machine.

5 Twist on the NUTRiBULLET blade and blend until smooth.

CHEF'S NOTE
Feel free to add more coconut milk or water for your desired consistency.

SWEET SPINACH & BANANA SMOOTHIE

Ingredients

FIBRE+

- 2 handfuls spinach
- 1 banana
- 1 carrot
- 4 tbsp low fat natural yogurt
- 1 tbsp honey
- Handful of ice cubes

Method

1 Rinse the spinach and the carrot well. Roughly chop the carrot and remove any thick stalks from the spinach.

2 Peel the banana and break into three pieces.

3 Add all the ingredients to the NUTRiBULLET tall cup, making sure they do not go past the MAX line on your machine.

4 Twist on the NUTRiBULLET blade and blend until smooth.

CHEF'S NOTE
Add more yoghurt to suit your own taste making sure you keep below the MAX line.

AVOCADO, BANANA & KIWI SMOOTHIE

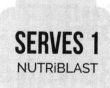

Ingredients

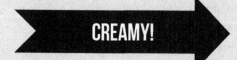

CREAMY!

- 1 handful spinach
- ½ avocado
- 1 banana
- 1 kiwi
- 300ml/10½floz almond milk
- ¼ tsp ground cinnamon
- Handful of ice cubes

Method

1 Rinse the spinach and remove any thick stalks.

2 Halve, stone and peel the avocado. Peel the banana and break into three pieces.

3 Peel the kiwi and halve.

4 Add all the ingredients to the NUTRiBULLET tall cup. Make sure they do not go past the MAX line on your machine.

5 Twist on the NUTRiBULLET blade and blend until smooth.

CHEF'S NOTE
Kiwi is also one of the few foods rich in vitamin B6, which supports the immune system.

CLEMENTINE & SPINACH CHIA SMOOTHIE

Ingredients

LACTOSE FREE

- 1 handful spinach
- 3 seedless clementines
- 1 banana
- 120ml/4floz soya milk
- 1 tbsp chai seeds
- Water

Method

1 Rinse the spinach well, removing any thick stalks.

2 Peel the clementines. Peel the banana and break into three pieces.

3 Add all the ingredients to the NUTRiBULLET tall cup, making sure they do not go past the MAX line on your machine. Add water if you want to alter the consistency.

4 Twist on the NUTRiBULLET blade and blend until smooth.

CHEF'S NOTE
A little added organic honey or agave nectar makes this a sweet treat breakfast smoothie.

BLUEBERRY BLAST

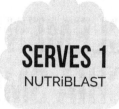

SERVES 1
NUTRiBLAST

Ingredients

- 1 handful fresh blueberries
- 1 handful kale
- 1 handful spinach
- 1 banana
- ½ carrot
- ½ lemon
- 1 tbsp flax seeds
- Water

Method

1 Wash the blueberries, kale, spinach. Wash, top & tail the carrot.

2 Remove any thick stalks from the kale and spinach.

3 Peel the banana and break into three pieces.

4 Add all the ingredients to the NUTRiBULLET tall cup, making sure they do not go past the MAX line on your machine.

5 Twist on the NUTRiBULLET blade and blend until smooth.

CHEF'S NOTE
The strong fibre, antioxidant and anti-inflammatory content of flaxseed is great for healthy smoothies.

ALMOND BUTTER VANILLA SMOOTHIE

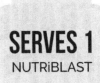

Ingredients

- 1 pear
- 200ml/7floz unsweetened almond milk
- 1 handful spinach
- 2 tbsp of oats

- 1 tbsp almond butter
- ¼ tsp vanilla extract
- Handful of ice cubes

Method

1 Rinse the spinach and pear.

2 Core the pear and remove any thick stalks from the spinach.

3 Add all the ingredients to the NUTRiBULLET tall cup, making sure they do not go past the MAX line on your machine.

4 Twist on the NUTRiBULLET blade and blend until smooth.

CHEF'S NOTE
Packed with goodness this breakfast smoothie will slowly release energy throughout the morning to help keep you energised.

STRAWBERRY & ALMOND BUTTER SMOOTHIE

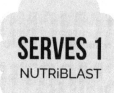

Ingredients

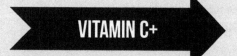

VITAMIN C+

- 200ml/7floz almond milk
- 4 strawberries
- ½ banana
- 2 handfuls collared greens
- 1 tbsp flax seeds
- 1 tbsp almond butter
- Handful of ice cubes

Method

1 Rinse the strawberries and greens.

2 Peel the banana.

3 Add all the ingredients to the NUTRiBULLET tall cup, making sure they do not go past the MAX line on your machine.

4 Twist on the NUTRiBULLET blade and blend until smooth.

CHEF'S NOTE
Add more strawberries to suit your taste or try a handful of raspberries too.

Skinny

NUTRiBULLET

DETOX & CLEANSE SMOOTHIES

SUPER-CLEANSING SMOOTHIE

Ingredients

- 1 handful spinach
- 1 handful romaine leaves
- ¼ cucumber
- 1 celery stalk
- 1 pear
- 1 banana

- 250ml/8 floz coconut water
- 4 fresh mint leaves
- ½ lemon
- 1 tbsp chia seeds
- 1cm/½ inch fresh ginger root, peeled

Method

1 Rinse the ingredients well.

2 Core the pear. Peel the banana. Peel and de-seed the lemon.

3 Add all the ingredients to the NUTRiBULLET tall cup. Make sure they do not go past the MAX line on your machine.

4 Twist on the NUTRiBULLET blade and blend until smooth.

CHEF'S NOTE
Spice it up with a pinch of cayenne, cinnamon and turmeric.

GRAPEFRUIT & SPINACH SMOOTHIE

Ingredients

CLEANSING!

- 1 grapefruit
- 1 handful seedless green grapes
- ½ banana
- 1 handful spinach
- 1cm/½ inch fresh ginger root, peeled
- 1 date
- Water

Method

1 Rinse the grapes and the spinach well; remove any thick stalks from the spinach

2 Peel and de-seed grapefruit. Peel the banana and stone the date.

3 Add all the ingredients to the NUTRiBULLET tall cup, making sure they do not go past the MAX line on your machine.

4 Twist on the NUTRiBULLET blade and blend until smooth.

CHEF'S NOTE
The date will add a subtle natural sweetness to this smoothie.

APPLE & KALE SMOOTHIE

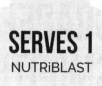

SERVES 1
NUTRiBLAST

Ingredients

DIETARY FIBRE

- 1 handful kale
- 1 apple
- 250ml/8½ floz coconut water
- Handful of ice cubes

Method

1 Rinse the kale and the apple well.

2 Remove any thick stalks from the kale and core the apple

3 Add to the NUTRiBULLET tall cup, along with the coconut water. Make sure the ingredients don't go past the MAX line on your machine.

4 Twist on the NUTRiBULLET blade and blend until smooth.

CHEF'S NOTE
Kale is packed with fibre and sulphur, both great for detoxifying your body and keeping your liver healthy.

SIMPLE SPINACH & SPICE SMOOTHIE

Ingredients

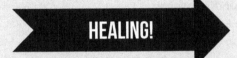

HEALING!

- 2cm/1 inch fresh ginger root
- ½ - 1 tsp ground cinnamon
- 2 handfuls spinach
- Water

Method

1 Rinse the spinach well and remove any thick stalks.

2 Peel and grate the ginger.

3 Add all the ingredients to the NUTRiBULLET tall cup, making sure they do not go past the MAX line on your machine.

4 Twist on the NUTRiBULLET blade and blend until smooth.

CHEF'S NOTE
Ginger is thought to cleanse the body by stimulating digestion, circulation and sweating.

PEAR & GINGER FLAX SMOOTHIE

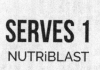

Ingredients

NATURALLY SWEET!

- 1 pear
- 1 handful spinach
- 1 tbsp flax seeds
- 1 tsp coconut oil
- 2cm/1 inch fresh ginger root
- 2 tsp honey
- Water

Method

1 Rinse the pear and the spinach and remove any thick stalks from the spinach.

2 Core the pear. Peel & grate the ginger.

3 Add everything to the NUTRiBULLET tall cup. Make sure you don't go past the MAX line on your machine.

4 Twist on the NUTRiBULLET blade and blend until smooth.

CHEF'S NOTE
Flax seeds are thought to help eliminate the toxins from the body, normalize the metabolism, reduce blood sugar level and regulate appetite.

GREEN & FRUITY JUICE

Ingredients

- ¼ cucumber
- 1 handful spinach
- ½ avocado
- 1 celery stalk

- 2 sprigs mint
- 1 kiwi
- ½ apple
- Water

Method

1 Rinse the ingredients well and remove any thick stalks from the spinach.

2 Halve and stone the avocado. Peel the kiwi fruit. Core the apple.

3 Add all the ingredients to the NUTRiBULLET tall cup, making sure they do not go past the MAX line on your machine.

4 Twist on the NUTRiBULLET blade and blend until smooth.

CHEF'S NOTE

Raw spinach is rich in glutathione that is helpful to overall well-being.

SPINACH, MINT & GINGER JUICE

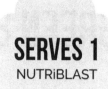

SERVES 1
NUTRiBLAST

Ingredients

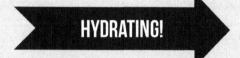

HYDRATING!

- 1 handful spinach
- 1 handful fresh mint
- 1 tbsp lemon juice
- ½ cucumber
- 4 celery stalks
- 2cm/1 inch fresh ginger root
- Water

Method

1 Rinse the ingredients well and remove any thick stalks from the spinach.

2 Peel and grate the ginger.

3 Add all the ingredients to the NUTRiBULLET tall cup, making sure they do not go past the MAX line on your machine.

4 Twist on the NUTRiBULLET blade and blend until smooth.

CHEF'S NOTE
The hydration properties of cucumber along with the lemon juice create a cleansing effect that helps to clear out the digestive system.

WINTER SMOOTHIE

Ingredients

- 1 apple
- 1 pear
- 1 handful fresh cranberries
- 2cm/1 inch fresh ginger root

- 3 large kale leaves
- 1 handful shredded green cabbage
- Water

Method

1 Wash the ingredients well.

2 Core the apple and pear. Peel and grate the ginger.

3 Add the ingredients to the NUTRiBULLET tall cup, making sure they do not go past the MAX line on your machine.

4 Twist on the NUTRiBULLET blade and blend until smooth.

CHEF'S NOTE
There is some evidence that cranberries may be linked to a reduced risk of kidney stones, cardiovascular disease and cancer.

CARROT, PEAR & BROCCOLI SMOOTHIE

Ingredients

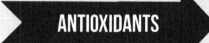

ANTIOXIDANTS

- 1 carrot
- ½ pear
- 200g/7oz broccoli florets
- Water

Method

1 Rinse the ingredients well.

2 Core the pear. Nip the ends off the carrot.

3 Combine all the ingredients in the NUTRiBULLET tall cup. Make sure they don't go past the MAX line on your machine.

4 Twist on the NUTRiBULLET blade and blend until smooth.

CHEF'S NOTE
Broccoli has a number of outstanding health properties, including high concentrations of essential vitamins & fibre.

Skinny

NUTRiBULLET

DIGESTIVE HEALTH SMOOTHIES

PINEAPPLE & PARSLEY SMOOTHIE

Ingredients

- ½ fresh pineapple
- ½ banana
- 120ml/4 floz water
- 120ml/4 floz coconut water

- A few sprigs fresh parsley
- 1 handful spinach
- ¼ avocado
- 1 tsp freshly grated ginger root

Method

1 Pour the water and coconut water into the NUTRiBULLET tall cup.

2 Peel the pineapple & banana and add to the cup.

3 Peel and stone the avocado. Give the parsley and spinach a rinse, and add to the cup, along with the grated ginger.

4 Make sure the ingredients do not go past the MAX line on your machine.

5 Twist on the NUTRiBULLET blade and blend until smooth.

CHEF'S NOTE
Ginger helps improve digestion, prevents bloating and decreases intestinal gas.

CORIANDER & GINGER SMOOTHIE

Ingredients

- 1 handful fresh coriander
- 1 cucumber
- 3 tbsp lime juice
- 1-inch peeled fresh ginger root
- ¼ fresh pineapple
- 1 tomato
- Water

Method

1 Rinse the coriander, cucumber and tomato.

2 Roughly chop the cucumber, halve the tomato and peel the pineapple.

3 Add all the ingredients to the NUTRiBULLET tall cup, making sure they do not go past the MAX line on your machine.

4 Twist on the NUTRiBULLET blade and blend until smooth.

CHEF'S NOTE

Coriander has been used to treat stomach disorders in traditional Chinese medicine throughout the ages.

BLUEBERRY & SPINACH SMOOTHIE

Ingredients

DIGESTION BOOSTER

- 1 handful blueberries
- 2 handfuls spinach
- ½ tbsp ground flax seeds
- 120ml/½ cup coconut milk
- Water

Method

1 Rinse the blueberries and the spinach well.

2 Add all the ingredients to the NUTRiBULLET tall cup, making sure they do not go past the MAX line on your machine. Add a little water if needed to take it to the line (or a little more coconut water)

3 Twist on the NUTRiBULLET blade and blend until smooth.

CHEF'S NOTE
Ground flax seeds are a good source of soluble fibre - which is essential to aid healthy digestion.

SOOTHING GREEN FRUIT SMOOTHIE

Ingredients

- 1 handful shredded romaine, or green leaf lettuce
- 1 handful spinach
- 1 slice of fennel bulb
- ¼ apple
- ¼ pear
- 1 small handful fresh mint
- 1 small handful fresh coriander
- 1 tbsp lemon juice
- Water

Method

1 Rinse the ingredients well.

2 Remove any thick stalks from the spinach. Core the apple and pear,

3 Add all the ingredients to the NUTRiBULLET tall cup, making sure they do not go past the MAX line on your machine.

4 Twist on the NUTRiBULLET blade and blend until smooth.

CHEF'S NOTE

In Germany, coriander is officially approved for the treatment of mild gastrointestinal upsets, and to help stimulate the appetite.

CABBAGE, PINEAPPLE & PAPAYA SMOOTHIE

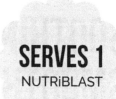

Ingredients

TOXIN CLEANSER

- ¼ pineapple
- ¼ papaya
- 1 handful shredded cabbage
- 1 handful spinach
- 200ml/7floz coconut water

Method

1 Wash the cabbage & spinach.

2 Peel the pineapple & papaya (don't worry about the seeds).

3 Add everything to the tall cup making sure they do not go past the MAX line on your machine.

4 Twist on the NUTRiBULLET blade and blend until smooth.

CHEF'S NOTE
Coconut water is thought to aid digestion by helping to eliminate body waste and release toxins.

GREEN CHIA SMOOTHIE

Ingredients

- 2 tbsp natural Greek yoghurt
- 1 handful spinach
- 1 handful kale
- 2 tbsp chia seeds
- ½ cucumber
- ½ apple
- 1 tbsp lemon juice
- A few fresh mint leaves

Method

1 Rinse the spinach, kale, cucumber, apple and mint.

2 Roughly chop the cucumber, core the apple and remove any thick stalks from the spinach & kale.

3 Combine all the ingredients in the NUTRiBULLET tall cup, making sure they do not go past the MAX line on your machine.

4 Twist on the NUTRiBULLET blade and blend until smooth.

CHEF'S NOTE

The ancient Aztecs long promoted the health benefits of chia seeds as a remedy for constipation.

FRUIT & GINGER SMOOTHIE

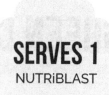

Ingredients

PROTEIN RICH

- 1 handful collared greens
- ½ avocado
- ½ banana
- 1 inch/2cm piece fresh ginger root
- 200g/7oz pineapple
- 120ml/4floz coconut water
- 120ml/4floz water

Method

1 Rinse the collared greens and remove any thick stalks.

2 Pour the coconut water into the NUTRiBULLET tall cup.

3 Halve and stone the avocado. Peel the banana, ginger root and pineapple and add to the cup.

4 Pour in the water, making sure not to go past the MAX line on your machine.

5 Twist on the NUTRiBULLET blade and blend until smooth.

CHEF'S NOTE
The fibre content of collard greens makes this cruciferous vegetable a natural choice for digestive system support.

GREEN KEFIR SMOOTHIE

Ingredients

PROBIOTICS

- 360ml/12½floz coconut water kefir
- 1 handful fresh pea shoots
- 1 handful fresh spinach
- 1 celery stalk
- 1 carrot

Method

1 Rinse the ingredients well.

2 Remove any thick stalks from the spinach and nip the ends off the carrot.

3 Add everything to the NUTRiBULLET tall cup, making sure they do not go past the MAX line on your machine.

4 Twist on the NUTRiBULLET blade and blend until smooth.

CHEF'S NOTE
Coconut Water Kefir is a naturally fermented beverage made from young coconuts. If you can't buy kefir just use regular coconut water.

CABBAGE & HONEY SMOOTHIE

Ingredients

AIDS DIGESTION

- 2 handfuls shredded green cabbage
- 2 tbsp lemon juice
- 1 tbsp organic honey
- Water

Method

1 Rinse the cabbage well and put them in the NUTRiBULLET tall cup.

2 Add the rest of the ingredients, making sure they don't go past the MAX line on your machine.

3 Twist on the NUTRiBULLET blade and blend until smooth.

CHEF'S NOTE

This smoothie is good for general intestinal health. Drink twice a day to combat constipation problems.

FRUITY HEMP SMOOTHIE

SERVES 1

NUTRiBLAST

Ingredients

- 1 banana
- 1 handful strawberries
- 1 handful spinach
- 2 tbsp hulled hemp seeds

- 1 tbsp pea powder protein
- 200ml/7 floz coconut water
- 1 tsp agave nectar

Method

1 Peel the banana and break into three pieces.

2 Rinse the spinach and strawberries well.

3 Add all the ingredients to the NUTRiBULLET tall cup, making sure they do not go past the MAX line on your machine.

4 Twist on the NUTRiBULLET blade and blend until smooth.

CHEF'S NOTE
Hemp seeds aid digestion, balance hormones and improve metabolism.

SOYA KIWI SMOOTHIE

Ingredients

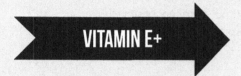

VITAMIN E+

- 1 handful kale
- 2 celery stalks
- 1 pear
- 2 kiwi fruits
- 200ml/7floz soya milk

Method

1 Rinse the kale, celery and pear.

2 Core the pear and peel the kiwifruits.

3 Add all the ingredients to the NUTRiBULLET tall cup, making sure they do not go past the MAX line on your machine.

4 Twist on the NUTRiBULLET blade and blend until smooth.

CHEF'S NOTE
Kiwis are believed to contain a unique compound which helps to digest the proteins found in red meat.

Skinny

NUTRiBULLET

ENERGY BOOST SMOOTHIES

MATCHA AND PEAR SMOOTHIE

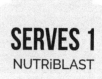

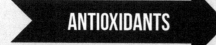

Ingredients

- 1 handful spinach
- 1 pear
- ½ tsp matcha green tea powder
- 300ml/10½ floz unsweetened almond milk
- Water

Method

1 Rinse the spinach and pear. Core the pear and remove any hard stalks from the spinach.

2 Add all the ingredients to the NUTRiBULLET tall cup, making sure they do not go past the MAX line on your machine.

3 Top up with a little water if needed.

4 Twist on the NUTRiBULLET blade and blend until smooth.

CHEF'S NOTE
Matcha is powdered green tea leaves. Because whole leaves are ingested, it's a more potent source of goodness than steeped green tea.

GREEN AVOCADO & COCONUT SMOOTHIE

Ingredients

- ½ avocado
- 1 handful kale
- ½ apple
- 1 handful spinach
- 250ml/8½ floz coconut water
- 4 fresh mint leaves
- Water

Method

1 Wash the kale, spinach, mint and apple. Cut any thick stems from the kale and spinach.

2 Core the apple. Peel and stone the avocado.

3 Add all the ingredients to the NUTRiBULLET tall cup. Make sure they do not go past the MAX line on your machine.

4 Top up with a little water if needed.

5 Twist on the NUTRiBULLET blade and blend until smooth.

CHEF'S NOTE
Avocados are rich in monosaturated fats. These are good fats that your body uses to create energy quickly.

GREEN FRUIT SMOOTHIE

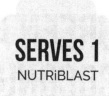

Ingredients

NUTRIENT DENSE

- ½ cucumber
- 1 stalk celery
- 1 handful kale
- 1 apple
- 1 pear
- 1 tsp lemon juice
- Water

Method

1 Rinse the ingredients well.

2 Core the apple and pear. Remove any thick stalks from kale.

3 Add all the ingredients to the NUTRiBULLET tall cup, finishing with a little water, but make sure not to pass the MAX line on your machine.

4 Twist on the NUTRiBULLET blade and blend until smooth.

CHEF'S NOTE
Kale is a real energy booster that provides the essential minerals of copper, potassium, iron and phosphorus.

ORANGE AND SPINACH SMOOTHIE

Ingredients

ESSENTIAL FATS →

- 1 orange
- ½ banana
- 1 handful spinach
- 120ml/4floz coconut water
- 1 tbsp hemp seeds
- Water

Method

1 Rinse the spinach and remove any thick stalks.

2 Peel and de-seed the orange.

3 Peel the banana.

4 Add all the ingredients to the NUTRiBULLET tall cup. Make sure they do not go past the MAX line on your machine.

5 Twist on the NUTRiBULLET blade and blend until smooth.

CHEF'S NOTE
Containing essential omega-3 fats, hemp seeds provide long sustaining energy.

APPLE & SPINACH SMOOTHIE

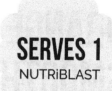

Ingredients

ENERGY BOOST

- 2 apples
- 1 handful seedless green grapes
- 1 handful spinach
- 1 kiwi
- ½ cucumber
- Water

Method

1 Rinse the apple, grapes, greens and cucumber.

2 Core the apples.

3 Peel the kiwifruit and cut it in two.

4 Roughly chop the greens and cucumber

5 Add all the ingredients to the NUTRiBULLET tall cup, making sure they do not go past the MAX line on your machine.

6 Twist on the NUTRiBULLET blade and blend until smooth.

CHEF'S NOTE
Spinach is extremely high in magnesium and plays a vital role in producing energy.

LEMON GREEN BLAST

Ingredients

- 5 celery stalks
- 1 handful of kale
- 1 handful of spinach
- 1 handful flat-leaf parsley
- 1 lemon
- 1 cucumber
- Water

Method

1 Rinse the ingredients well.

2 Remove any thick stalks from the kale and spinach.

3 Peel and de-seed the lemon. Roughly chop the cucumber.

4 Add all the ingredients to the NUTRiBULLET tall cup. Make sure they don't go past the MAX line on your machine.

5 Twist on the NUTRiBULLET blade and blend until smooth.

CHEF'S NOTE

Parsley contains lots of vitamin C that boosts cell regeneration and helps the body stay energised.

COCONUT & FLAX SMOOTHIE

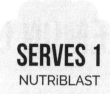

Ingredients

GOOD FATS

- 250ml/8½floz coconut water
- ½ pear
- ½ avocado
- 1 handful spinach
- 1 tbsp flax seeds
- Water

Method

1 Wash the spinach and the pear.

2 Remove any thick stalks from the spinach and core the pear.

3 Peel and stone the avocado.

4 Add all the ingredients except the water to the NUTRiBULLET tall cup, making sure they do not go past the MAX line on your machine.

5 Twist on the NUTRiBULLET blade and blend until smooth. Add water a little at a time and reblend until it reaches your desired consistency to drink.

CHEF'S NOTE
Flaxseeds are one of the richest sources of vital Omega-3 fatty acids.

SPINACH & STRAWBERRY SMOOTHIE

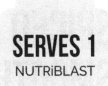

Ingredients

ENERGY +

- 2 handfuls spinach
- 1 apple
- 1 banana
- 5 strawberries
- ½ orange
- Water

Method

1 Rinse the spinach, apple and strawberries.

2 Core the apple. Peel the banana and break into three pieces.

3 Peel and de-seed the orange.

4 Add all the ingredients to the NUTRiBULLET tall cup, making sure they do not go past the MAX line on your machine.

5 Twist on the NUTRiBULLET blade and blend until smooth.

CHEF'S NOTE
Bananas boost energy by slowly releasing carbs into the bloodstream as glucose.

SPICED PERSIMMON SMOOTHIE

Ingredients

VITAMIN RICH →

- 250ml/8½ floz almond milk
- 1 persimmon
- 1 handful spinach
- ½ tsp cinnamon
- ¼ tsp cardamom
- 1 date
- Water

Method

1 Wash the persimmon and the spinach. Cut the persimmon into quarters.

2 Halve and stone the date. Remove any thick stalks from the spinach.

3 Add all the ingredients to the NUTRiBULLET tall cup, making sure they do not go past the MAX line on your machine.

4 Top up with a little water if needed.

5 Twist on the NUTRiBULLET blade and blend until smooth.

CHEF'S NOTE
Persimmons have a high vitamin and mineral content including vitamins A, C, E and B6, as well as dietary fiber, manganese, copper, magnesium, potassium, and phosphorous.

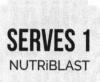

SWEET & SPICY GREEN SMOOTHIE

Ingredients

- 1 handful kale
- 1 apple
- ½ lemon
- 2cm/1 inch slice peeled fresh ginger root

- ¼ tsp cayenne pepper
- 1 tbsp organic honey
- Water

Method

1 Rinse the kale and apple.

2 Remove any thick stalks from the kale. Core the apple. Peel and de-seed the lemon.

3 Add all the ingredients to the NUTRiBULLET tall cup, making sure they do not go past the MAX line on your machine.

4 Twist on the NUTRiBULLET blade and blend until smooth.

CHEF'S NOTE
Eating 'good carbs' such as honey during a workout helps your muscles stay nourished longer and delays fatigue.

KALE & KIWI BLAST

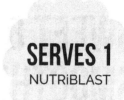
Ingredients

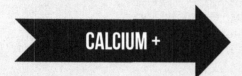

CALCIUM +

- 2 handfuls kale
- 2 kiwis
- 1 orange
- 2 tsp lemon juice
- Water

Method

1 Rinse the kale and remove any thick stalks

2 Peel the kiwi fruits and cut them in half.

3 Peel and de-seed the orange.

4 Add all the ingredients to the NUTRiBULLET tall cup. Making sure they do not go past the MAX line on your machine.

5 Twist on the NUTRiBULLET blade and blend until smooth.

CHEF'S NOTE
High in vitamins and minerals, kale is a great energy booster and key source of calcium.

Skinny

NUTRiBULLET
SMOOTHIES FOR SKIN

SWISS CHARD & GRAPE SMOOTHIE

Ingredients

- 2 handfuls Swiss chard
- 1 handful green seedless grapes
- 1 pear
- 1 orange
- 2 bananas
- 1 tsp chia seeds
- Water
- Ice

Method

1 Rinse the fruit and vegetables well.

2 Remove the stems from the chard and roughly chop the leaves.

3 Core the pear. Peel and de-seed the orange. Peel the bananas and break each into three pieces.

4 Add the fruit, vegetables, chia seeds and water to the NUTRiBULLET tall cup. Add ice to taste, making sure you don't pass the MAX line on your machine.

5 Twist on the NUTRiBULLET blade and blend until smooth.

CHEF'S NOTE
The antioxidants in grapes can help increase blood circulation; leading to healthy and glowing skin.

ALMOND KALE SMOOTHIE

Ingredients

CLEANSING →

- 250ml/8½ floz unsweetened almond milk
- 1 handful kale leaves
- 1 banana
- 1 tbsp natural peanut butter
- Ice to taste

Method

1 Rinse the kale and cut off any thick stalks.

2 Peel the banana and break into three pieces.

3 Add the ingredients to the NUTRiBULLET tall cup. Add ice to taste, making sure you don't pass the MAX line on your machine.

4 Twist on the NUTRiBULLET blade and blend until smooth.

CHEF'S NOTE
The sulphur and fibre in kale aid the body's detox.

PROTEIN BLAST

Ingredients

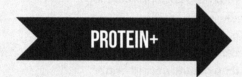

PROTEIN+

- 120ml/4floz coconut water
- 2 handfuls kale
- 300g/11oz fresh pineapple
- 1 banana
- 1 scoop organic vanilla protein powder
- Handful of ice

Method

1 Rinse the kale well and remove any thick stalks.

2 Peel and roughly chop the pineapple.

3 Peel the banana and break into three pieces.

4 Add the ingredients to the NUTRiBULLET tall cup. Making sure the ice doesn't go past the MAX line on your machine.

5 Twist on the NUTRiBULLET blade and blend until smooth.

CHEF'S NOTE
Use more coconut water and less ice if you prefer.

KALE & MANGO SMOOTHIE

Ingredients

GLOWING SKIN

- 1 handful kale
- ½ mango
- 2 stalks celery
- 1 tbsp fresh flat-leaf parsley
- Water

Method

1 Rinse the kale, celery and parsley.

2 Peel & stone the mango.

3 Add all the ingredients to the NUTRiBULLET tall cup. Make sure they don't go past the MAX line on your machine.

4 Twist on the NUTRiBULLET blade and blend until smooth.

CHEF'S NOTE

Vitamin A rich kale is excellent for skin and eyesight.

SPINACH & SWEET POTATO SMOOTHIE

Ingredients

BETA CAROTENES

- 1 banana
- 1 handful spinach
- 1 small sweet potato (cooked)
- 300ml/10½floz unsweetened almond milk
- Handful of ice

Method

1 Rinse the spinach well and remove any thick stalks.

2 Peel the banana and break into three pieces.

3 Add all the ingredients to the NUTRiBULLET tall cup, adding a few ice cubes to taste. Make sure you do not pass the MAX line on your machine.

4 Twist on the NUTRiBULLET blade and blend until smooth.

CHEF'S NOTE
Almond milk is high in vitamin E, which is essential to your skin's health.

AVOCADO & COCONUT SMOOTHIE

Ingredients

HEART HEALTHY

- 300ml/10½ floz coconut water
- 1 handful spinach
- 2 kiwis
- ½ avocado

Method

1 Rinse the spinach well and remove any thick stalks.

2 Peel the kiwis and cut them in half. Peel & stone the avocado.

3 Add all the ingredients to the NUTRiBULLET tall cup. Make sure they do not go past the MAX line on your machine.

4 Twist on the NUTRiBULLET blade and blend until smooth.

CHEF'S NOTE
Avocados are rich in healthy fatty acids, vitamins and antioxidants that can improve your skin from the inside.

KALE, KIWI & CORIANDER SMOOTHIE

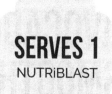

Ingredients

DIETARY FIBRE →

- 1 handful kale
- 2 kiwis
- 1 orange
- 2 tbsp fresh coriander/cilantro
- 1 stalk celery
- Water

Method

1 Rinse the kale, coriander and celery. Remove any thick stalks from the kale.

2 Peel the kiwis and orange, de-seed the orange.

3 Add everything to the NUTRiBULLET tall cup making sure not to go past the MAX line on your machine.

4 Twist on the NUTRiBULLET blade and blend until smooth.

CHEF'S NOTE
Kiwi contains several skin friendly nutrients including vitamin C, E and antioxidants.

COCONUT, APPLE & GINGER SMOOTHIE

SERVES 1
NUTRiBLAST

Ingredients

- ½ romaine lettuce
- ½ apple
- ¼ cucumber
- ¼ avocado

- ½ lemon
- 2cm/1inch piece peeled fresh ginger
- 250ml/8½floz coconut water

Method

1 Rinse the lettuce, apple, cucumber and parsley.

2 Core the apple. Peel & stone the avocado. Peel & de-seed the lemon.

3 Add all the ingredients to the NUTRiBULLET tall cup, making sure they do not go past the MAX line on your machine.

4 Twist on the NUTRiBULLET blade and blend until smooth.

CHEF'S NOTE

Ginger contains around forty antioxidant properties that prevent free radical damage and protect against aging.

WINTER GREEN SMOOTHIE

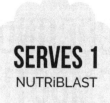

SERVES 1
NUTRiBLAST

Ingredients

ANTIOXIDANT NUTRIENTS

- 1 carrot
- ½ orange
- 1 handful spinach
- 4 broccoli florets
- 1 banana
- 1 apple

Method

1 Rinse the spinach, broccoli & apple. Remove any thick stalks from the spinach.

2 Peel the orange and banana. Core the apple, peel & de-seed the orange.

3 Add all the ingredients to the NUTRiBULLET tall cup, making sure they do not go past the MAX line on your machine.

4 Twist on the NUTRiBULLET blade and blend until smooth.

CHEF'S NOTE
The presence of dietary fibre, vitamins, minerals and antioxidants in broccoli are beneficial to skin.

MINT TEA BLAST

Ingredients

- 120ml/4 floz chilled mint tea
- 1 handful baby spinach
- ½ romaine lettuce
- 5 leaves mint
- 1 lemon
- 1 tsp honey
- Water

Method

1 Rinse the spinach, lettuce and mint.

2 Peel and de-seed the lemon.

3 Add everything to the NUTRiBULLET tall cup.
Make sure the ingredients do not go past the MAX
line on your machine.

4 Twist on the NUTRiBULLET blade and blend until
smooth.

CHEF'S NOTE
Lettuce is a rich source of vitamin A.
Vitamin A increases cell turnover which in
turn helps to revitalize your skin.

KEFIR SPINACH BLAST

Ingredients

PROBIOTIC GOODNESS

- 1 handful baby spinach
- ½ cucumber
- ½ avocado
- 1 kiwi
- 1 orange
- 120ml/4floz kefir
- Water

Method

1 Rinse the spinach & cucumber.

2 Peel and stone the avocado. Peel and de-seed the orange.

3 Roughly chop the cucumber. Halve, peel and stone the avocado.

4 Peel the kiwi.

5 Add all the ingredients to the NUTRiBULLET tall cup, making sure they do not go past the MAX line on your machine.

6 Twist on the NUTRiBULLET blade and blend until smooth.

CHEF'S NOTE
Kefir contains lactic acid that is an anti-aging ingredient.

Skinny

NUTRiBULLET

CLEAN & GREEN SMOOTHIES

VEGETABLE & CITRUS BLAST

SERVES 1
NUTRiBLAST

Ingredients

- 1 handful spinach
- ¼ cucumber
- 2 sticks of celery
- A few sprigs fresh parsley
- A few mint leaves
- 1 large carrot

- 1 apple
- 2 orange seedless segments
- 2 tbsp lime juice
- Water

Method

1 Rinse the ingredients well.

2 Remove any thick stalks from the spinach, core the apple and nip the ends off the carrot.

3 Combine all the ingredients in the NUTRiBULLET tall cup, adding water to no farther than the MAX line on your machine.

4 Twist on the NUTRiBULLET blade and blend until smooth.

CHEF'S NOTE
If you prefer a thinner drink, you might want to add more water after blending.

TROPICAL GREEN SMOOTHIE

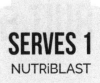

Ingredients

- 2 handfuls spinach
- 175ml/6floz unsweetened almond milk
- ½ small banana
- 200g/7oz fresh pineapple,

- 2 pitted dates
- ½ - 1 tsp ground cinnamon
- Ice cubes to taste

Method

1 Rinse the spinach and remove any thick stalks.

2 Peel the banana and pineapple.

3 Halve and pit the dates

4 Add all the ingredients to the NUTRiBULLET tall cup. Make sure they do not go past the MAX line on your machine.

5 Twist on the NUTRiBULLET blade and blend until smooth.

CHEF'S NOTE
Use as much almond milk as you need to fill to the max.

FRUIT & LEAVES

Ingredients

- 1 romaine lettuce
- 3 sticks celery
- 1 handful spinach
- 1 apple
- 1 pear
- 1 banana
- 1 tbsp lemon juice
- Water

Method

1 Rinse the ingredients well. Snap the celery and remove any thick stalks from the spinach.

2 Core the apple and pear, but don't peel them. Peel the banana and break into three.

3 Add all the ingredients to the NUTRiBULLET tall cup. Make sure they do not go past the MAX line on your machine.

4 Twist on the NUTRiBULLET blade and blend until smooth.

CHEF'S NOTE
Add coriander and parsley for extra health and flavour!

PAPAYA SMOOTHIE

Ingredients

GREEN POWER

- 150g/5oz papaya
- 1 handful kale
- 1 handful spinach
- ½ banana
- ½ green apple
- 4 tbsp water

Method

1 Rinse the spinach, kale and apple.

2 Peel the papaya and the banana; break the banana into three pieces.

3 Core the apple and cut the half in two.

4 Add all the ingredients to the NUTRiBULLET tall cup. Make sure they do not go past the MAX line on your machine.

5 Twist on the NUTRiBULLET blade and blend until smooth.

CHEF'S NOTE
If the mixture is too thick for your taste, add water and re-blend, making sure to stay below the MAX line.

MANGO & COCONUT SMOOTHIE

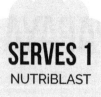

Ingredients

PROTECTS HEALTH

- 1 mango
- ½ lime
- ½ banana
- 2 handfuls kale
- 200ml/7floz light coconut milk

Method

1 Rinse the ingredients well.

2 Remove any thick stalks from the kale.

3 Add the coconut milk to the NUTRiBULLET tall cup.

4 Peel and stone the mango. Peel and de-seed the lime. Peel the banana and break into three pieces.

5 Add everything to the cup making sure the ingredients do not go past the MAX line on your machine.

6 Twist on the NUTRiBULLET blade and blend until smooth.

CHEF'S NOTE
Try with spinach or other chard instead of kale.

ORANGE & SWEET POTATO SMOOTHIE

Ingredients

INCREASES ENERGY

- 1 orange
- 100g/3½oz sweet potato
- 3 handfuls kale
- 2 tbp chia seeds
- Water

Method

1 Rinse the kale and remove any thick stalks.

2 Peel and de-seed the orange.

3 Add all the ingredients to the cup making sure they do not go past the MAX line on your machine.

4 Twist on the NUTRiBULLET blade and blend until smooth.

CHEF'S NOTE
Sweet potatoes are a good source of potassium, dietary fibre & niacin.

STRAWBERRY & BASIL SMOOTHIE

Ingredients

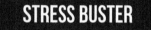

- Handful strawberries
- Handful fresh basil leaves
- 1 tbsp chia seeds
- 1 banana
- 2 handfuls spinach
- 200ml/7floz almond milk

Method

1 Pour the almond milk into the NUTRiBULLET tall cup.

2 Wash the strawberries, basil and spinach.

3 Peel the banana and break into three pieces.

4 Add all the ingredients to the cup making sure they do not go past the MAX line on your machine.

5 Twist on the NUTRiBULLET blade and blend until smooth.

CHEF'S NOTE
Basil is an excellent source of vitamin K and manganese.

GRAPE & SPINACH BLAST

Ingredients

NATURALLY SWEET

- 1 handful seedless green grapes
- 100g/3½oz pineapple
- 2 handfuls spinach
- ½ banana
- Water
- Ice cubes

Method

1 Rinse the grapes and the spinach well.

2 Peel the pineapple & banana and add to the NUTRiBULLET tall cup.

3 Add the water and some ice cubes, making sure the ingredients do not go past the MAX line on your machine.

4 Twist on the NUTRiBULLET blade and blend until smooth.

CHEF'S NOTE
Experiment with the quantities of water and ice to make your smoothie the consistency you like best.

VERY GREEN SMOOTHIE

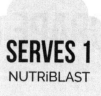

SERVES 1
NUTRiBLAST

Ingredients

GREEN GOODNESS

- 2 handfuls kale
- ½ cucumber
- 3 celery sticks
- ½ lemon or lime
- 1 apple
- Water

Method

1 Rinse the ingredients well. Remove any thick stalks from the kale.

2 Core the apple.

3 Add everything to the NUTRiBULLET tall cup making sure the ingredients do not go past the MAX line on your machine.

4 Twist on the NUTRiBULLET blade and blend until smooth.

CHEF'S NOTE
Try with a little fresh ginger blended with the smoothie to add kick!

MOJITO SMOOTHIE

Ingredients

AIDS DIGESTION

- 1 handful spinach
- 6-8 fresh mint leaves
- 200ml/7floz coconut water
- 3 tbsp lime juice
- 1 banana
- Ice cubes

Method

1 Rinse the spinach and mint well.

2 Peel the banana and break into three pieces.

3 Add all the ingredients to the NUTRiBULLET tall cup, making sure they do not go past the MAX line on your machine.

4 Twist on the NUTRiBULLET blade and blend until smooth.

CHEF'S NOTE
If you have a sweet tooth add a teaspoon of organic honey or agave nectar before blending.

ALMOND & STRAWBERRY SMOOTHIE

Ingredients

- 1 handful spinach
- 1 handful kale
- 3 sprigs fresh parsley
- 1 handful strawberries
- 1 tbsp fresh lemon juice
- ¼ cucumber
- 200ml/7floz unsweetened almond milk

Method

1 Rinse the ingredients well.

2 Remove any thick stalks from the spinach & kale.

3 Add all the ingredients to the NUTRiBULLET tall cup. Make sure they do not go past the MAX line on your machine.

4 Twist on the NUTRiBULLET blade and blend until smooth.

CHEF'S NOTE
Almond milk is low in fat, but high in energy, proteins, lipids and fibre. It also contains calcium, iron, magnesium, phosphorus, potassium, sodium, and zinc.

WHEATGRASS POWER SMOOTHIE

Ingredients

- 1 banana
- ½ grapefruit
- ¼ avocado
- 1 handful each kale & spinach
- 1-inch peeled fresh root ginger
- 1 tsp wheatgrass powder
- Water

Method

1 Rinse the kale and spinach well and remove any thick stalks.

2 Peel and de-seed the grapefruit. Peel and stone the avocado. Peel the banana and break into three pieces.

3 Add all the ingredients to the NUTRiBULLET tall cup making sure they do not go past the MAX line on your machine.

4 Twist on the NUTRiBULLET blade and blend until smooth.

CHEF'S NOTE

Sometimes referred to as a 'fountain of youth' wheatgrass has outstanding nutritional values, Packed with vitamins, minerals, amino acids and enzymes.

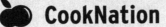 **CookNation**

Other
COOKNATION
TITLES

If you enjoyed 'The *Skinny* NUTRiBULLET Super Green Smoothies Recipe Book' you may also be interested in other *Skinny* NUTRiBULLET titles by CookNation.

Visit **www.bellmackenzie.com** to browse the full catalogue.

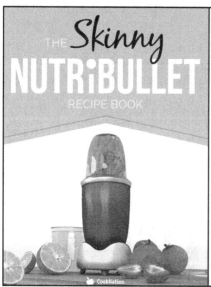

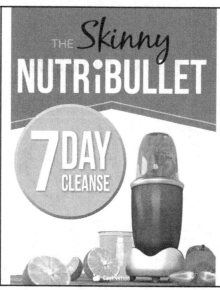

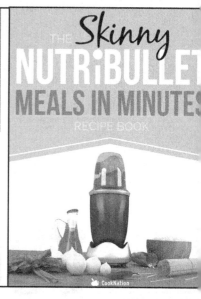

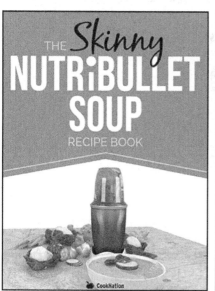

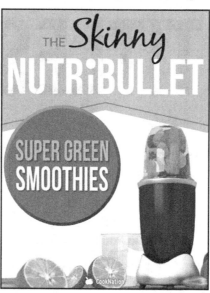

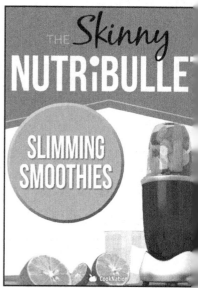

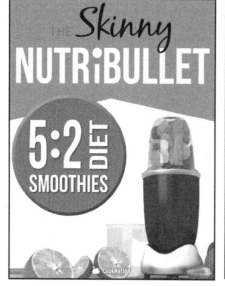

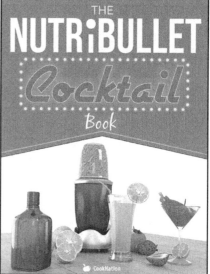

Made in the USA
Middletown, DE
12 December 2019